MW00951000

YOUR GUIDE TO
Living Well With Heart Disease

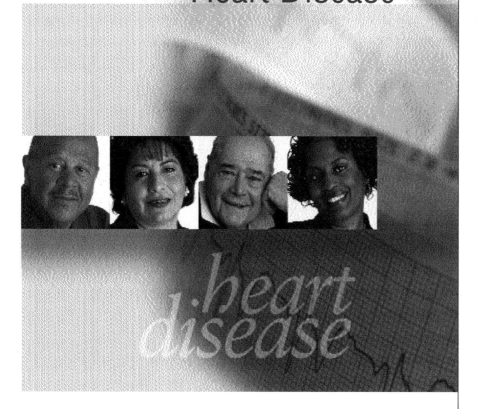

.heart
disease

U.S. DEPARTMENT OF HEALTH AND HUMAN SERVICES
National Institutes of Health
National Heart, Lung, and Blood Institute

NIH Publication No. 06–5270
November 2005

Written by: Marian Sandmaier

U.S. DEPARTMENT OF HEALTH AND HUMAN SERVICES
National Institutes of Health
National Heart, Lung, and Blood Institute

Contents

Introduction

Chances are, you're reading this book because you or someone close to you has heart disease. Perhaps your doctor has recently told you that you have a heart condition, and you're looking for information on how to take good care of yourself. Perhaps you've known about your condition for some time and are interested in the latest knowledge on treatment and self-care. Perhaps you've recently had a heart attack or heart surgery and want some guidance on making the best possible recovery.

This book will address all of these concerns. It is a step-by-step guide to helping people with heart disease make decisions that will protect and improve their heart health. It will give you information about lifestyle habits, medicines, and other treatments that can lessen your chances of having a heart attack—either a first attack or a repeat one. If you have already had a heart attack or have undergone a heart procedure, you will find guidance on how to recover well, both physically and emotionally.

But this book is not just about preventing and treating problems. It is also about how to live well with heart disease. It will help you to make decisions that allow you to live as fully, healthfully, and enjoyably as possible, even as you cope with the demands of your heart condition. As you read this book, you will find that caring for your heart and caring for yourself are deeply inter-twined. To find out why and how, read on.

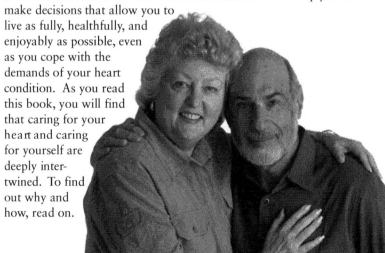

Heart Disease:
A Wakeup Call

If you have heart disease, you may understandably hope that it's only a temporary ailment, one that can be cured with medicine or surgery. But heart disease is a lifelong condition: Once you have it, you'll always have it. It's true that procedures such as angioplasty and bypass surgery can help blood and oxygen flow more easily through the coronary arteries that lead to the heart. But the arteries remain damaged, which means that you're more likely to have a heart attack. It is sobering, yet important, to realize that the condition of your blood vessels will steadily worsen unless you make changes in your daily habits. Many people die of complications from heart disease, or become permanently disabled. That's why it is so vital to take action to control this serious condition.

The good news is that you can control heart disease. There is much you can do to manage your heart condition, reduce your risk of a first or repeat heart attack, and improve your chances of living a long, rewarding life. The sooner you get started, the better your chances of avoiding further heart problems, feeling better, and staying well. So use this handbook to find out more about your own heart condition and what you can do to improve it. You have the power to make a positive difference in your heart health—and you can start making that difference today.

3

WILBUR "MAC" MCCOTTRY

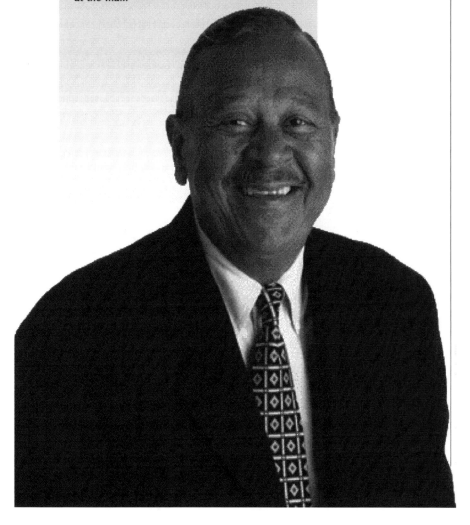

"My real wakeup call came about 2 weeks after my heart bypass operation. The doctor said he did all he could to save my life and the rest was up to me. Well, those words shook me up. I knew exactly what he meant: lose the weight, quit smoking, exercise more, and make changes to my diet. So I took it very, very seriously. I lost 70 lbs. I am walking 2 miles three times a week in a program at the mall."

What Is Heart Disease?

Coronary heart disease is the main form of heart disease. It occurs when the coronary arteries, which supply blood to the heart muscle, become hardened and narrowed due to a buildup of plaque on the arteries' inner walls. Plaque is the accumulation of cholesterol, fat, and other substances. As plaque continues to build up in the arteries, blood flow to the heart is reduced.

Coronary heart disease—often simply called heart disease—can lead to a heart attack. A heart attack happens when a cholesterol-rich plaque bursts and releases its contents into the bloodstream. This causes a blood clot to form over the plaque, totally blocking blood flow through the artery and preventing vital oxygen and nutrients from getting to the heart. A heart attack can cause permanent damage to the heart muscle.

Heart disease includes a number of other serious conditions, including:

Angina. More than 6 million Americans live with angina, which is chest pain or discomfort that occurs when the heart muscle is not getting enough blood. The inadequate blood flow is caused by narrowed coronary arteries, due to an accumulation of plaque. A bout of angina is not a heart attack, but it means that you're more likely to have a heart attack than someone who doesn't have angina. There are two kinds of angina:

Stable angina has a recognizable pattern. It may feel like pressure or a squeezing pain in your chest. The pain may also occur in your shoulders, arms, neck, jaw, or back. It may also feel like indigestion. Stable angina pain is generally brought on by some kind of exertion or strain (such as climbing stairs or experiencing emotional stress), and it is usually relieved by rest or medicine.

Unstable angina is more serious than stable angina. Occurring at any time, unstable angina often reflects a change in a previously stable pattern of angina. Episodes of unstable angina are usually more frequent, painful, and longer lasting than bouts of stable angina, and a re less often relieved by rest or medicine. Unstable angina is a sign that you may have a heart attack very soon. The symptoms are the same as if you are having a heart attack. (See page 46 for heart attack warning signs.) If you have any of these symptoms, you should call 9–1–1 right away so that you can get immediate treatment.

Congestive heart failure. Congestive heart failure is a life-threatening condition in which the heart cannot pump enough blood to supply the body's needs. Affecting nearly 5 million Americans, heart failure occurs when excess fluid collects in the body as a result of heart weakness or injury. This condition leads to a buildup of fluid in the lungs, causing swelling of the feet, tiredness, weakness, and breathing difficulties.

High blood pressure is the leading cause of congestive heart failure in the United States. Heart disease and diabetes are also major underlying causes of heart failure. People who have had a heart attack are at high risk of developing this condition.

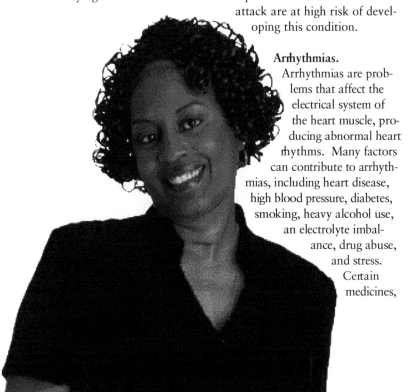

Arrhythmias. Arrhythmias are problems that affect the electrical system of the heart muscle, producing abnormal heart rhythms. Many factors can contribute to arrhythmias, including heart disease, high blood pressure, diabetes, smoking, heavy alcohol use, an electrolyte imbalance, drug abuse, and stress. Certain medicines, dietary supplements, and herbal remedies also cause arrhythmias in some people.

A common type of arrhythmia is called **atrial fibrillation,** a disorder affecting 2.2 million Americans. It is more common in older people and those with certain inborn heart problems. Atrial fibrillation occurs when the heart's two upper chambers (the atria) quiver instead of beating normally. Blood isn't pumped completely out of these chambers, making it more likely to pool and clot. If a clot leaves the heart and becomes lodged in an artery in the brain, a stroke results. About 15 percent of strokes occur in people with atrial fibrillation.

Another type of arrhythmia called **ventricular fibrillation** occurs when the lower heart chambers (the ventricles) quiver, preventing the heart from effectively pumping blood. This is the most dangerous type of heart rhythm disturbance. To prevent collapse and sudden cardiac death, it is vital to get immediate emergency medical help for ventricular fibrillation.

Getting Tested for Heart Disease

You may be reading this book because you think you might have heart disease but aren't yet sure. Keep in mind that heart disease doesn't always announce itself with symptoms. That means you could have heart disease and still feel perfectly fine. The best course is to talk with your doctor about your personal degree of heart disease risk and about whether getting tested is a good idea.

Most screening tests for heart disease are done outside of the body and are painless. After taking a careful medical history and doing a physical examination, your doctor may give you one or more of the following tests:

Electrocardiogram (ECG or EKG) makes a graph of the heart's electrical activity as it beats. This test can show abnormal heart-beats, heart muscle damage, blood flow problems in the coronary arteries, and heart enlargement.

Stress test (or treadmill test or exercise ECG) records the heart's electrical activity during exercise, usually on a treadmill or exercise bike. If you are unable to exercise due to arthritis or another health condition, a stress test can be done without exercise. Instead, you can take a medicine that increases blood flow to the heart muscle and shows whether there are any problems in that flow.

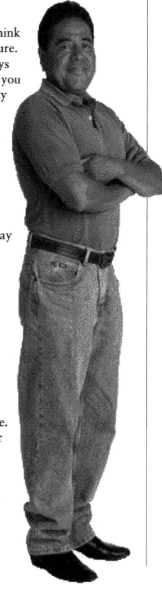

Nuclear scan (or thallium stress test) shows the working of the heart muscle as blood flows through the heart. A small amount of radioactive material is injected into a vein, usually in the arm, and a camera records how much is taken up by the heart muscle.

Echocardiography changes sound waves into pictures that show the heart's size, shape, and movement. The sound waves also can be used to see how much blood is pumped out by the heart when it contracts.

Coronary angiography (or angiogram or arteriography) shows an x ray of blood flow problems and blockages in the coronary arteries. A thin, flexible tube called a catheter is threaded through an artery of an arm or leg up into the heart. A dye is then injected into the tube, allowing the heart and blood vessels to be filmed as the heart pumps. The picture is called an angiogram or arteriogram.

Ventriculogram is frequently a part of the x-ray dye test described before. It is used to get a picture of the heart's main pumping chamber, typically the left ventricle.

Intracoronary ultrasound uses a catheter that measures blood flow. It creates a picture of the coronary arteries that shows the thickness and other features of the artery wall. This lets the doctor see blood flow and any blockages.

In addition, several new, highly sensitive screening tests have been developed. Ask your doctor about these tests:

Carotid doppler ultrasound uses sound waves to detect blockages and narrowing of the carotid artery in the neck, both of which can signal an increased risk for heart attack or stroke.

Electron-beam computed tomography is a superfast scan that provides a snapshot of the calcium buildup in your coronary arteries.

Should You Get a Heart Test at the Local Mall?

Recent media attention has raised public interest in the "total body scan" or "virtual scan," now offered at many malls around the country. This is a computed tomography (CT) scan that quickly screens for a number of diseases, including heart disease. Is the total body scan a good way to find out whether you have a heart condition?

Probably not. One of the problems with many mall-based body scans is that they use types of CT scanners known as spiral or helical. Neither of these types of scanners has proven effective for heart imaging. Furthermore, some spiral scanners transmit relatively high doses of radiation.

A CT heart scan should be performed using the U.S. Food and Drug Administration-approved, electron-beam CT scanner, which is lower in radiation. This type of scanner is available primarily in hospitals and other traditional health care settings. Getting tested in a medical setting also allows your doctor to interpret the results for you and evaluate your need for further testing.

It can pick up heart disease before you feel any symptoms. While promising, this test is not foolproof and requires careful evaluation by your doctor. (See "Should You Get a Heart Test at Your Local Mall?" above.)

Magnetic resonance imaging (MRI) is a scan using magnets and computers to create high-quality images of the heart's structure and functioning. It is often used to evaluate congenital heart disease. The test can also detect severe blockages in coronary arteries in people who are having unstable angina or a heart attack, thereby allowing immediate treatment to restore blood flow to the heart.

Controlling Your Risk Factors

If you have heart disease, you may wonder *why* you have it. The answer is that many personal characteristics, health conditions, and lifestyle habits can contribute to heart disease. These are called risk factors.

But risk factors do more than simply contribute to heart problems. They also increase the chances that existing heart disease will worsen. Since you already have heart disease, it is very important to find out about all of your risk factors and take active steps to control them.

Certain risk factors, such as getting older, can't be changed. Starting at age 45, a man's risk of heart disease begins to rise, while a woman's risk begins to increase at age 55. Family history of early heart disease is another risk factor that can't be changed. If your father or brother had a heart attack before age 55, or if your mother or sister had one before age 65, you are more likely to develop heart disease yourself.

While certain risk factors can't be changed, it's important to realize that you do have control over many others. Regardless of your age or family history, or how serious your heart disease is, you can take steps to reduce your risk of a first or repeat heart attack. You can also manage other problems associated with heart disease, such as angina, heart failure, and arrhythmias.

It may be tempting to believe that doing just one healthy thing will be enough to control heart disease. For example, you may hope that if you walk or swim regularly, you can still eat a lot of fatty foods and stay safe. Not so. To reduce your risk of a heart attack and other complications, it is vital to make changes that address each risk factor you have. You can make the changes gradually, one at a time. But making them is very important.

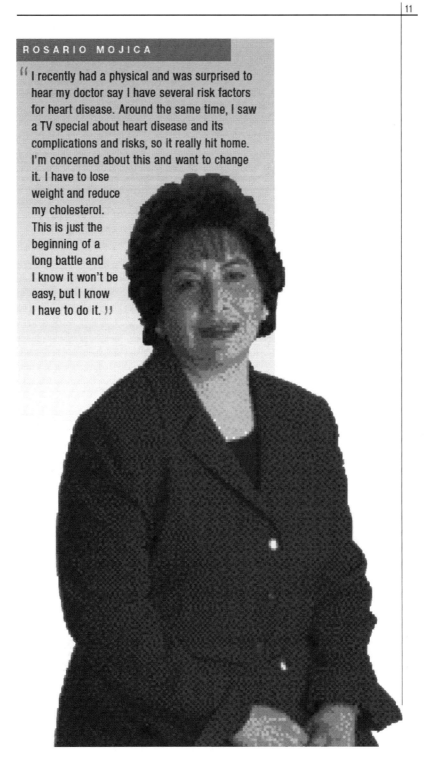

ROSARIO MOJICA

"I recently had a physical and was surprised to hear my doctor say I have several risk factors for heart disease. Around the same time, I saw a TV special about heart disease and its complications and risks, so it really hit home. I'm concerned about this and want to change it. I have to lose weight and reduce my cholesterol. This is just the beginning of a long battle and I know it won't be easy, but I know I have to do it."

While each risk factor may contribute to worsened heart disease, the more risk factors you have, the higher your risk. That's because risk factors tend to "gang up" and worsen each other's effects. For example, if you have high blood cholesterol and diabetes, your heart attack risk increases enormously. The message is clear: If you have heart disease, you must take immediate steps to reduce your risk of life-threatening medical problems. It's your heart and you have everything to gain from taking good care of it.

You and Your Doctor: A Healthy Partnership

Your doctor can be an important partner in helping you manage heart disease. He or she may already have spoken with you about your heart disease risk factors, but if not, be sure to ask about how to control all of them to help prevent future problems. Here are some tips for establishing good, clear communication with your doctor.

Speak up. Tell your doctor that you want to keep your heart disease from getting worse and would like help in achieving that goal. Ask questions about your chances of having a first heart attack or a repeat heart attack, your risk of other heart complications, and ways to lower those risks. If you haven't done so already, ask for tests that will determine your personal risk factors.

Be open. When your doctor asks you questions, answer them as honestly and fully as you can. While certain topics may seem quite personal, discussing them openly can help your doctor work with you more effectively to manage your heart condition.

Keep it simple. If you don't understand something your doctor says, ask for an explanation in plain language. Be especially sure you understand how to make the lifestyle changes your doctor recommends, as well as why and how to take each medication you're given. If you're worried about under- standing what the

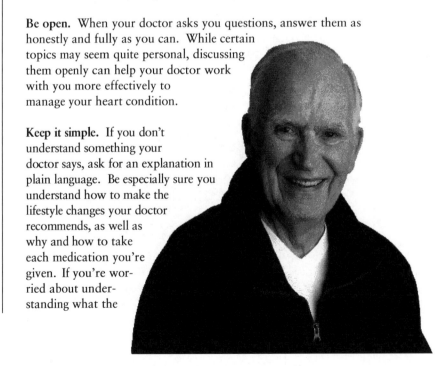

doctor says, or if you have trouble hearing, bring a friend or relative with you to your appointment. You may want to ask that person to write down the doctor's instructions for you.

Major Risk Factors

A strong partnership with your doctor is an important first step in managing heart disease. But to make a lasting difference, you'll also need to learn more about the kinds of habits and conditions that can worsen heart disease and what you can do about them. What follows is a guide to major risk factors for heart disease, heart attack, and other heart problems, and steps you can take to control or eliminate them.

Smoking

Smoking is the "leading cause of preventable death and disease in the United States," according to the Centers for Disease Control and Prevention. If you have heart disease and continue to smoke, your risk of having a heart attack is very high. If you live or work with others, your "secondhand" smoke can cause them numerous health problems, including a higher risk of heart attack—even if they don't smoke themselves. By the same token, if you have heart disease and live or work with someone who smokes, your own risk of heart attack goes up considerably.

Smoking puts stress on the heart in many ways. The nicotine in cigarettes constricts the coronary arteries, which raises blood pressure and forces the heart to work harder. Smoking also raises carbon monoxide levels and reduces oxygen levels in the blood. It's a double whammy: Smoking both increases the heart's need for oxygen and restricts the amount of oxygen it receives.

There is simply no safe way to smoke. Low-tar and low-nicotine cigarettes do not lessen the risks of a heart attack. The only safe and healthful course is not to smoke at all.

The good news is that quitting smoking will immediately and significantly reduce your risk of further heart disease complications. After a few days, once nicotine and carbon monoxide are cleared from your body, your blood pressure will go down and the levels of oxygen and carbon monoxide in your blood can return to normal. Within 1 year after quitting, your blood flow and breathing will be improved and your coughing and shortness of breath will be reduced.

Some people prefer to quit on their own, while others find group support helpful. A number of free or low-cost programs are available to help people stop smoking. They include classes offered by local chapters of the American Lung Association and the American Cancer Society. Other low-cost programs can be found through hospitals, health maintenance organizations (HMOs), workplaces, and community groups.

Also consider using a medicine that can help you stay off cigarettes. Some medications contain very small amounts of nicotine, which can help to lessen the urge to smoke. They include nicotine gum (available over the counter), a nicotine patch (available over the counter and by prescription), a nicotine inhaler (by prescription only), and a nicotine nasal spray (by prescription only). Another quitting aid is Bupropion SR, a medicine that contains no nicotine but reduces the craving for cigarettes. It is available only by prescription. While all of these medications can help people quit smoking, they are not safe for everyone. Talk with your doctor about whether you should try any of these medicines.

High Blood Pressure

High blood pressure, also known as hypertension, is another major risk factor for heart disease and heart attack. For those who already have heart disease, high blood pressure raises heart attack risk even higher. Hypertension also raises the risks of stroke, congestive heart failure, and kidney disease.

Blood pressure is the amount of force exerted by the blood against the walls of the arteries. Everyone has to have some blood pressure, so that blood can get to all of the body's organs. Blood pressure is usually expressed as two numbers, such as 120/80, and is measured in millimeters of mercury (mmHg).

The first number is the systolic blood pressure, the amount of force produced when the heart beats. The second number, or diastolic blood pressure, is the pressure that exists in the arteries between heartbeats. The higher your blood pressure, the harder your heart has to work, and the more "wear and tear" on your blood vessels.

High blood pressure is often called the silent killer because it usually doesn't cause symptoms. According to a national survey, two-thirds of people with high blood pressure do not have it under control.

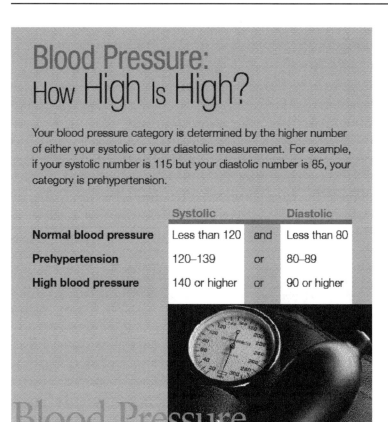

Blood Pressure:
How High Is High?

Your blood pressure category is determined by the higher number of either your systolic or your diastolic measurement. For example, if your systolic number is 115 but your diastolic number is 85, your category is prehypertension.

	Systolic		Diastolic
Normal blood pressure	Less than 120	and	Less than 80
Prehypertension	120–139	or	80–89
High blood pressure	140 or higher	or	90 or higher

Blood Pressure

But you can take action to control high blood pressure, and thereby avoid many life-threatening disorders.

Your health care provider should check your blood pressure on several different days before deciding whether it is too high. Blood pressure is considered high when it stays at or above 140/90 over a period of time. However, if you have diabetes, it is important to keep your blood pressure below 130/80.

For those with heart disease, it is especially important to control blood pressure to reduce the risks of stroke and heart attack. Even if you don't have high blood pressure, it is important to avoid developing prehypertension, a condition that increases your risk for high blood pressure.

Be aware, too, that a high systolic blood pressure level (first number) is dangerous. If your systolic blood pressure is 140 or higher (or 130 or higher if you have diabetes), you are more likely to develop heart disease complications and other problems even if your diastolic blood pressure (second number) is in the normal range. High systolic blood pressure is high blood pressure. If you have this condition, you will need to take steps to control it. High blood pressure can be controlled in two ways: by changing your lifestyle and by taking medication.

Changing your lifestyle. If your blood pressure is not too high, you may be able to control it entirely by losing weight if you are overweight, getting regular physical activity, limiting the salt in your food, cutting down on alcohol, and changing your eating habits. A special eating plan called DASH can help to lower blood pressure. DASH stands for Dietary Approaches to Stop Hypertension. The DASH eating plan emphasizes fruits, vegetables, whole-grain foods, and low-fat dairy products. It is rich in magnesium, potassium, calcium, protein, and fiber, but low in saturated fat, *trans* fat, total fat, and cholesterol. (*Trans* fat is a harmful type of dietary fat that forms when vegetable oil is hardened.) The diet also limits red meat, sweets, and sugar-containing beverages.

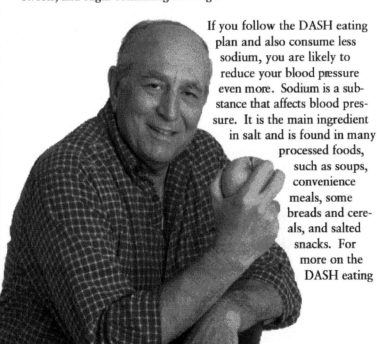

If you follow the DASH eating plan and also consume less sodium, you are likely to reduce your blood pressure even more. Sodium is a substance that affects blood pressure. It is the main ingredient in salt and is found in many processed foods, such as soups, convenience meals, some breads and cereals, and salted snacks. For more on the DASH eating

Sudden Symptoms:
Learn the Warning Signs of a Stroke

A stroke is a loss of blood flow to the brain that causes brain tissue to die. Stroke is a medical emergency. If you or someone you know has a stroke, it is important to recognize the symptoms so that you can get to a hospital quickly. Getting treatment within 60 minutes can prevent disability. The chief warning signs of a stroke are:

- Sudden numbness or weakness of the face, arm, or leg (especially on one side of the body).
- Sudden confusion, trouble speaking, or understanding speech.
- Sudden trouble seeing in one or both eyes.
- Sudden trouble walking, dizziness, or loss of balance or coordination.
- A sudden, severe headache with no known cause.

If you think someone might be having a stroke, call 9–1–1 immediately. Also, be sure that family members and others close to you know the warning signs of stroke. Give them a copy of this list.

Ask them to call 9–1–1 right away if you or someone else shows any signs of a stroke.

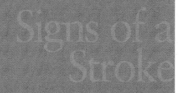
Signs of a Stroke

plan and other changes you can make to lower and prevent high blood pressure, see the National Heart, Lung, and Blood Institute's (NHLBI's) Web page, Your Guide to Lowering High Blood Pressure, which is listed in the "To Learn More" section of this guidebook.

Taking medication. If your blood pressure remains high even after you make lifestyle changes, your doctor will probably prescribe medicine. Depending on your health needs, your doctor may prescribe medication from the start, along with changes in your living habits. One recent study found that diuretics (water pills) work better than newer drugs to treat high blood pressure in many people. Other research shows that using a diuretic can reduce the risk of death from heart and blood vessel diseases, especially among people with diabetes. Talk with your doctor about making one of your high blood pressure medications a diuretic.

Keep in mind that lifestyle changes will help the medicine work more effectively. In fact, if you are successful with the changes you make in your daily habits, you may be able to gradually reduce the amount of medication you take.

Taking medicine to lower blood pressure can reduce your risk of heart attack, stroke, congestive heart failure, and kidney disease. Be sure to take your blood pressure medicine exactly as your doctor has prescribed it. Before you leave your physician's office, make sure you understand the amount of medicine you are supposed to take each day, and the specific times of day you should be taking it. If you take a drug and notice any uncomfortable side effects, ask your doctor about changing the dosage or switching to another type of medicine.

High Blood Cholesterol

The higher your blood cholesterol level, the greater your risk of having a heart attack. Because you have heart disease, your heart attack risk is already high, which means it is especially important to lower your cholesterol level. If you have diabetes as well as heart disease, your heart attack risk rises still higher. If you have both diseases, it is extremely important to take steps to keep both your cholesterol and your diabetes under control. Studies have proven that lowering cholesterol in people with heart disease reduces the risks for heart attack and death from heart disease and can actually prolong life.

How Cholesterol Causes Heart Problems
The body needs cholesterol to function normally. However, your body makes all the cholesterol it needs. Over time, extra cholesterol and fat circulating in the blood build up in the walls of the arteries that supply blood to the heart. This buildup, called plaque, makes the arteries narrower and narrower. If enough oxygen-rich blood cannot reach your heart, you may suffer chest pain, or angina. If the blood supply to a portion of the heart is completely cut off, the result is a heart attack. This usually happens when a cholesterol-rich plaque bursts, releasing the cholesterol into the bloodstream and causing a blood clot to form over the plaque.

Types of Cholesterol
Cholesterol travels in the blood in packages of fat (lipid) and protein called lipoproteins. Cholesterol packaged in low-density lipoprotein (LDL) is often called "bad" cholesterol, because too high a level of LDL in your blood can lead to blockages in your arteries. Another type of cholesterol is high-density lipoprotein (HDL) known as "good" cholesterol. That's because HDL helps to remove cholesterol from the body, preventing it from building up in your arteries.

Getting Tested
High blood cholesterol itself does not cause symptoms, so if your cholesterol level is too high, you may not be aware of it. So it is important to get your cholesterol levels checked regularly, especially if you have heart disease. A blood test called a "lipoprotein profile" measures the levels of all types of lipids, or fats, in your blood.

Total cholesterol is a measure of the cholesterol in all of your lipoproteins, including the bad cholesterol in LDL and the good cholesterol in HDL. Let's start with LDL levels. The higher your LDL number, the higher your risk of heart disease and heart attack. Knowing your LDL number is very important because it will determine the kind of treatment you may need. *The bottom line: If you have heart disease, reducing LDL cholesterol will reduce your risk of heart attack and can actually lengthen your life.*

Your HDL number tells a different story. The lower your HDL number, the higher your risk of heart disease and heart attack. Your lipoprotein profile test will also measure levels of triglycerides, which are another fatty substance in the blood.

HDL Cholesterol Level

An HDL cholesterol level of less than 40 mg/dL is a major risk factor for heart disease and heart attack. An HDL level of 60 mg/dL or higher is somewhat protective.

Your LDL Goal

The main goal of cholesterol-lowering treatment is to lower your LDL level enough to reduce your risk of heart attack. Reaching this goal is critically important if you have heart disease. The higher your risk category, the lower your LDL goal will be. For most people with heart disease or diabetes who are at high risk for heart attack, the goal of cholesterol-lowering treatment is an LDL level below 100 mg/dL.

If You Are in This Risk Category	Your LDL Goal
High risk	Is less than 100 mg/dL*
Very high risk	May be less than 70 mg/dL*

* Cholesterol levels are measured in milligrams (mg) of cholesterol per deciliter (dL) of blood.

Even Lower May Be Better

Because recent studies show a direct relationship between lower LDL cholesterol and reduced risk for heart attack, doctors now may prescribe more intensive cholesterol-lowering treatment for people at very high risk for a heart attack. For example, those with heart disease as well as diabetes, or those who have just had a heart attack, may have their LDL goal level lowered by their doctors to less than 70 mg/dL.

A Special Type of Risk

Nearly one-quarter of Americans have a group of risk factors known as metabolic syndrome. This condition is usually caused by over-weight or obesity, and by not getting enough physical activity. If you have heart disease, this cluster of risk factors greatly increases your risk of heart attack regardless of your LDL cholesterol level. You have metabolic syndrome if you have three or more of the following conditions:

- A waist measurement of 35 inches or more for a woman, and 40 inches or more for a man

What's Your Number?
Blood Cholesterol Levels for Preventing Heart Disease

Total Cholesterol Level	Category
Less than 200*	Desirable
200–239	Borderline high
240 and above	High

LDL Cholesterol Level	Category
Less than 100†	Optimal
100–129	Near optimal
130–159	Borderline high
160–189	High
190 and above	Very high

*All numbers refer to milligrams of cholesterol per deciliter (mg/dL) of blood.
† These cholesterol numbers and levels and goals are for the prevention of heart disease. If you already have heart disease, your LDL goal is less than 100 mg/dL. (See "Your LDL Goal" and "Even Lower May Be Better," page 20.)

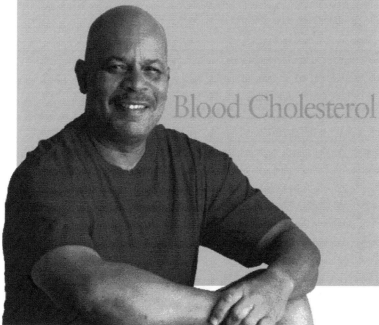

- Triglycerides of 150 mg/dL or more
- An HDL level of less than 50 mg/dL for a woman, and less than 40 mg/dL for a man
- Blood pressure of 130/85 mmHg or more (either number counts)
- Blood sugar of 100 mg/dL or more

If you have metabolic syndrome in addition to heart disease, your doctor will assess your risk factors and decide whether an LDL goal of less than 70 is right for you (especially if your triglycerides are 200 or higher, and your HDL is less than 40). You should make a particularly strong effort to reach and maintain your LDL goal. If you are overweight or obese, you will also need to take steps to lose weight by cutting back on high-calorie foods and increasing physical activity. Becoming physically active will help you correct the risk factors of the metabolic syndrome even if you don't need to lose weight.

How To Lower Your LDL
There are two main ways to lower your LDL cholesterol—through lifestyle changes alone, or through lifestyle changes combined with medication.

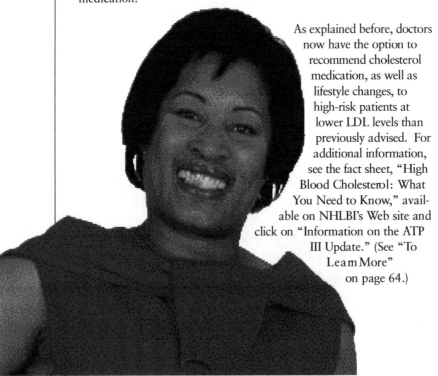

As explained before, doctors now have the option to recommend cholesterol medication, as well as lifestyle changes, to high-risk patients at lower LDL levels than previously advised. For additional information, see the fact sheet, "High Blood Cholesterol: What You Need to Know," available on NHLBI's Web site and click on "Information on the ATP III Update." (See "To Learn More" on page 64.)

Lifestyle changes. One important treatment approach is called TLC, which stands for Therapeutic Lifestyle Changes. This treatment helps to reduce LDL cholesterol through a diet that is low in saturated fat (the main dietary culprit that raises blood cholesterol), *trans* fat, and dietary cholesterol, as well as through regular physical activity and weight management.

Everyone who needs to lower LDL cholesterol should use this TLC program. Maintaining a healthy weight and getting regular physical activity are especially important for people who have metabolic syndrome. Adopt the TLC approach and you'll lower your chances of having a heart attack and other heart disease complications. Both the TLC eating plan and DASH eating plan recommend foods that are lower in saturated fats, *trans* fats, and cholesterol, such as vegetables and fruits, whole grains, low-fat milk products; and lean meats, fish, or poultry. The TLC plan simply puts more emphasis on decreasing saturated fat, *trans* fat, and cholesterol to lower blood cholesterol levels.

For a complete description of the TLC program, see the section on "Therapeutic Lifestyle Changes," available on NHLBI's Web site at www.nhlbi.nih.gov/chd/. This Web page also includes tips on shopping, cooking, and eating out for those who need to lower their cholesterol.

Medication. If your LDL level is above your goal, your doctor will prescribe medications at the same time you are making lifestyle changes. If you do need medication, be sure to use it along with the TLC approach. This will keep the dose of medicine as low as possible, and will lower your risk in other ways as well. You will also need to control all of your other heart disease risk factors, including high blood pressure, diabetes, and smoking.

Overweight and Obesity

If you have heart disease and are overweight or obese (extremely overweight), your risks of heart attack and other heart complications rise sharply. This is true even if you have no other risk factors. Being overweight or obese also increases your chances of developing other major risk factors for heart disease and heart attack, such as diabetes, high blood pressure, and high blood cholesterol. Overall, obese people are more likely to die of heart disease than normal-

Are You at a Healthy Weight?

Here is a chart for men and women that gives the BMI for various heights and weights*

BODY MASS INDEX

	21	22	23	24	25	26	27	28	29	30	31
4'10"	100	105	110	115	119	124	129	134	138	143	148
5'0"	107	112	118	123	128	133	138	143	148	153	158
5'1"	111	116	122	127	132	137	143	148	153	158	164
5'3"	118	124	130	135	141	146	152	158	163	169	175
5'5"	126	132	138	144	150	156	162	168	174	180	186
5'7"	134	140	146	153	159	166	172	178	185	191	198
5'9"	142	149	155	162	169	176	182	189	196	203	209
5'11"	150	157	165	172	179	186	193	200	208	215	222
6'1"	159	166	174	182	189	197	204	212	219	227	235
6'3"	168	176	184	192	200	208	216	224	232	240	248

*Weight is measured with underwear but not shoes.

What Does Your BMI Mean?

Categories:

Normal weight: BMI =18.5–24.9. Good for you! Try not to gain weight.

Overweight: BMI = 25–29.9. Do not gain any weight, especially if your waist measurement is high. You need to lose weight if you have two or more risk factors for heart disease and are overweight, or have a high waist measurement.

Obese: BMI = 30 or greater. You need to lose weight. Lose weight slowly—about 1/2 to 2 pounds a week. See your doctor or nutritionist if you need help.

Source: Clinical Guidelines on the Identification, Evaluation and Treatment of Overweight and Obesity in Adults: The Evidence Report; National Heart, Lung, and Blood Institute, in cooperation with the National Institute of Diabetes and Digestive and Kidney Diseases, National Institutes of Health; NIH Publication 98-4083; June 1998.

weight individuals. The bottom line: Maintaining a healthy weight is a necessary part of controlling heart disease.

Should You Choose To Lose?
Do you need to lose weight to help protect your heart? You can find out by taking these simple steps.

Step 1: Get your number. Take a look at the chart on page 24. You'll see that your weight in relation to your height gives you a number called a body mass index (BMI). A BMI from 18.5 to 24.9 indicates a normal weight. A person with a BMI from 25 to 29.9 is overweight, while someone with a BMI of 30 or higher is obese. Those in the overweight and obese categories have a higher risk of heart attack and other heart disease complications. The higher your BMI, the greater your risk.

Step 2: Take out a tape measure. The second step is to take your waist measurement. For women, a waist measurement of over 35 inches increases the risk of heart attack, as well as the risks of high blood pressure, diabetes, and other serious health conditions. For men, a waist measurement of more than 40 inches raises these risks. To measure your waist correctly, stand and place a tape measure around your middle, just above your hipbones. Measure your waist just after you breathe out.

Once you've taken these steps—found out your BMI and taken your waist measurement—you can use the information to decide whether you need to take off pounds. While you should talk with your doctor about whether you should lose weight, keep these guidelines in mind:

- If you have heart disease and are overweight or obese, you should lose weight.
- If you have heart disease and a high waist measurement (over 35 inches for a woman; over 40 inches for a man), you should lose weight.
- If you have two or more risk factors for heart disease and are overweight or obese, you should lose weight.
- If your weight and waist measurement are in the normal range, keep them that way! Avoid becoming overweight or adding extra inches around your middle.

Lose a Little, Win a Lot

If you need to lose weight, here's some good news: A small weight loss—just 5 to 10 percent of your current weight—can help to lower the risks of heart attack and other serious medical disorders. The best way to take off pounds is to do so gradually, by getting more physical activity and eating a balanced diet that is lower in calories and fat. For some people at very high risk, medication also may be necessary. To develop a weight-loss or weight-maintenance program that works well for you, consult with your doctor, registered dietitian, or qualified nutritionist. For ideas on how to lose weight safely and keep it off, see the section on "Aim for a Healthy Weight," available on NHLBI's Web site. (See "To Learn More" on page 64.)

Physical Inactivity

Many of us put off getting regular physical activity—and then put it off some more. But to protect our hearts, we must keep moving. For people with heart disease, physical inactivity greatly increases the risk of worsened disease. Lack of physical activity also contributes to other heart disease risk factors, such as high blood pressure, diabetes, and overweight.

Fortunately, research shows that as little as 30 minutes of moderate-intensity physical activity on most and preferably all days of the week helps to protect heart health. This level of activity can reduce your risk of heart disease complications, as well as lessen your chances of having a stroke, high blood pressure, diabetes, colon cancer, and other serious medical disorders.

Examples of moderate activity are taking a brisk walk, light weight-lifting, dancing, raking leaves, washing a car, housecleaning, or gardening. If you prefer, you can divide your 30-minute activity into shorter periods of at least 10 minutes each. If you have heart disease or another type of heart problem, be sure to see your doctor before starting a program of regular physical activity. To find out about easy, enjoyable ways to boost your activity level, see the "Guide to Physical Activity" page on NHLBI's Web site at: www.nhlbi.nih.gov/health/public/heart/obesity/lose_wt/phy_act.htm.

Diabetes

If you have diabetes, you have about the same high risk for heart attack as someone who has heart disease itself. Those who have heart disease and diabetes have an even higher risk for heart attack than those who have either heart disease or diabetes alone. Up to three-quarters of those who have diabetes die of some type of heart or blood vessel disease. However, if you have diabetes, there is much you can do to prevent the complications of this condition.

The type of diabetes that most commonly develops in adulthood is called type 2 diabetes. In this type of diabetes, the pancreas makes insulin but the body cannot use it properly and gradually loses the ability to produce it. Type 2 diabetes is a serious disease. In addition to increasing the risks for heart disease and heart attack, diabetes is the #1 cause of kidney failure, blindness, and lower limb amputation in adults. Diabetes can also lead to nerve damage, difficulties in fighting infection, and delayed wound healing.

A major risk factor for type 2 diabetes is overweight, especially having extra weight around the waist. Other risk factors include physical inactivity and a family history of diabetes. Type 2 diabetes is more common among American Indians, Hispanic Americans, Asian Americans, and Pacific Islanders. Women who have had diabetes during pregnancy (gestational diabetes), or who gave birth to a baby weighing more than 9 pounds, are also more likely to develop type 2 diabetes in later life.

Symptoms of diabetes may include fatigue, nausea, frequent urination, unusual thirst, weight loss, blurred vision, frequent infections, and slow healing of sores. But type 2 diabetes develops gradually and sometimes has no symptoms. In fact, nearly 6 million Americans who have this serious disease are not aware of it. Even if you have no symptoms, if you are overweight or have any other risk factors for type 2 diabetes, ask your doctor about getting tested for it. You have diabetes if your fasting blood glucose level is 126 mg/dL or higher.

If you have diabetes, controlling your blood glucose (blood sugar) levels will help to prevent complications. Because diabetes is so s t rongly linked with heart disease and heart attack, you must manage your diabetes very carefully. It is also especially important to control your blood pre s s u re and cholesterol levels. (See "The ABCs of Diabetes Control" on the next page.) Recommended levels of blood pre s s u re and blood cholesterol are lower for people with diabetes than for most others. Not smoking, getting regular physical activity, and taking aspirin daily (if your doctor recommends it) also are im po r ant ways to prevent heart disease complications if you have diabetes.

Some people do not yet have diabetes, but are at high risk for developing the disease. About 40 percent of Americans aged 40–74 have a condition known as prediabetes, where blood glucose levels are higher than normal but not yet in the diabetic range. Prediabetes is defined as a fasting blood glucose level of 100–125 mg/dL.

If you have heart disease and also have prediabetes, it is extremely important to improve your blood glucose levels in order to prevent the development of diabetes. The good news: A recent study shows that many people with prediabetes can prevent or delay diabetes by eating a lower fat, lower calorie diet and getting 30 minutes of moderate physical activity at least 5 days per week.

The ABCs of
Diabetes Control

If you have diabetes, three key steps can help you lower your risk of heart attack and stroke. Follow these ABCs:

A **is for A1C test,** which is short for hemoglobin A1C. This test measures your average blood glucose over the last 3 months. It lets you know if your blood glucose level is under control. Get this test at least twice a year. Number to aim for: below 7.

B **is for blood pressure.** The higher your blood pressure, the harder your heart has to work. Get your blood pressure measured at every doctor's visit. Numbers to aim for: below 130/80 mmHg.

C **is for cholesterol.** LDL, or "bad" cholesterol, builds up and clogs your arteries. Get your LDL cholesterol tested at least once a year. Number to aim for: below 100 mg/dL. If you have both diabetes and heart disease, your doctor may advise you to aim for a lower target number, for example, less than 70.

To lower your risk of heart attack and stroke, also take these steps:

- Follow your doctor's advice about getting physical activity every day.
- Eat less salt and sodium, saturated fat, *trans* fat, and cholesterol.
- Eat more fiber. Choose fiber-rich whole grains, fruits, vegetables, and beans.
- Stay at a healthy weight.
- If you smoke, stop.
- Take medicines as prescribed.
- Ask your doctor about taking aspirin.
- Ask others to help you manage your diabetes.

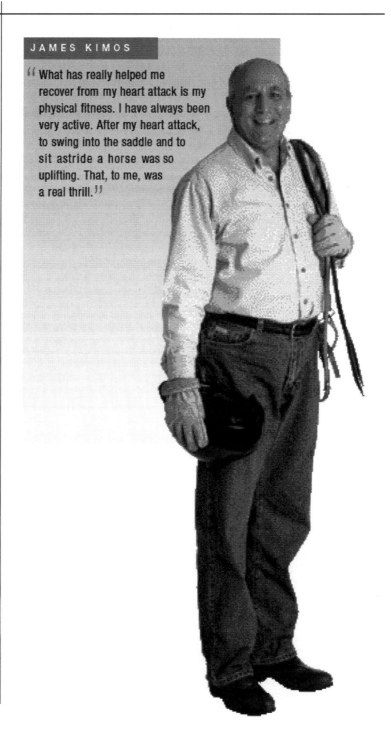

JAMES KIMOS

"What has really helped me recover from my heart attack is my physical fitness. I have always been very active. After my heart attack, to swing into the saddle and to sit astride a horse was so uplifting. That, to me, was a real thrill."

What Else Affects Heart Disease?

A number of other factors also contribute to heart disease, including certain health conditions, medicines, and other substances. Here is what you need to know:

Stress

Stress is linked to heart disease in a number of ways. Research shows that the most commonly reported "trigger" for a heart attack is an emotionally upsetting event, particularly one involving anger. In addition, some common ways of coping with stress, such as overeating, heavy drinking, and smoking are clearly bad for your heart.

The good news is that sensible health habits can have a protective effect. For people with heart disease, regular physical activity not only relieves stress but also can directly lower the risk of heart disease complications. Participating in a stress management program can help to prevent recurrent heart attacks and repeat heart procedures. Good relationships count, too. Developing strong personal ties can help to improve recovery after a heart attack.

Much remains to be learned about the connections between stress and heart disease, but a few things are clear. Staying physically active, developing a wide circle of supportive people in your life, and sharing your feelings and concerns with them can help you to be happier and live longer.

Alcohol

Recent research suggests that moderate drinkers are less likely to develop heart disease than people who don't drink any alcohol or who drink too much. Small amounts of alcohol may help protect against heart disease by raising levels of "good" HDL cholesterol.

If you are a nondrinker, this is not a recommendation to start drinking. Moreover, if you already have heart disease, you should be especially careful about using alcohol. Talk with your doctor about the impact of alcohol use on heart disease and other health conditions you may have. If you do decide to drink, moderation is the key. Moderate drinking is defined as no more than one drink per day for women, and no more than two drinks per day for men.

Heavy drinking is hazardous to your heart. More than three drinks per day can raise blood pressure. Meanwhile, binge drinking can contribute to stroke and doubles the risk of dying after a heart attack. Too much alcohol also can damage the heart muscle, leading to heart failure. Heavy drinking also raises the risk of developing metabolic syndrome, a cluster of heart disease risk factors that is particularly dangerous for people who already have heart disease.

Sleep Apnea

Sleep apnea is a serious disorder in which a person briefly and repeatedly stops breathing for short periods of time during sleep. People with untreated sleep apnea are more likely to have a heart attack, stroke, high blood pressure, and congestive heart failure.

Sleep apnea tends to develop in middle age, and men are twice as likely as women to have the condition. Other factors that increase risk are overweight and obesity, smoking, use of alcohol or sleeping pills, and a family history of sleep apnea. Symptoms include heavy snoring and gasping or choking during sleep, along with extreme daytime sleepiness.

If you think you might have sleep apnea, ask your doctor for a test called polysomnography, which is usually performed overnight in a sleep center. If you are overweight, even a small weight loss—10 percent of your current weight—can relieve mild cases of sleep apnea.

Other self-help treatments include quitting smoking and avoiding alcohol and sleeping pills. Sleeping on your side rather than on your back also may help. Some people benefit from a mechanical device that helps to maintain a regular breathing pattern by increasing air pressure through the nasal passages. For very serious cases, surgery may be needed.

Menopausal Hormone Therapy

Until recently, it was thought that menopausal hormone therapy could lower the risks of heart attack and stroke for women with heart disease. But research now shows that **women with heart disease should *not* take this medication.** Menopausal hormone therapy can involve the use of an estrogen-plus-progestin medicine or an estrogen-alone medicine. Studies on each type of medicine show that:

- Estrogen-plus-progestin medication increases the risk of heart attack during the first few years of use, and also increases the risks of stroke, blood clots, and breast cancer.
- Estrogen-only medication increases the risks of stroke and venous thrombosis (a blood clot that usually occurs in one of the deep veins of the legs). Estrogen-only medicine will not prevent heart attacks.

If you have heart disease and are currently taking or considering taking menopausal hormone therapy, talk with your doctor about safer medicines for controlling heart disease, for preventing osteoporosis, and/or for relieving menopausal symptoms.

C-Reactive Protein (CRP)

An elevated level of this blood protein is a sign of inflammation. Studies indicate that people with low CRP levels tend to have a slower progression of heart disease as well as fewer heart attacks and deaths from heart disease, than those with higher levels of the protein. Whether CRP plays a role in causing heart disease is not known.

A high-sensitivity CRP blood test can measure the level of this protein in your blood. Elevated levels can be lowered with the same statin medications that lower LDL cholesterol. Getting more physical activity, losing weight if you are overweight, eating a healthy diet, and quitting smoking will also reduce CRP levels.

Treatments for Heart Disease

If you have heart disease, you know by now that it's vital to control it. As emphasized before, making lifestyle changes that improve your risk factors is one important part of treatment. Eating well, getting regular physical activity, and maintaining a healthy weight will help to lessen the severity of your condition. If you smoke, you'll need to quit. Reducing stress and limiting alcohol use can also improve your heart health. And if you have diabetes, you will need to carefully manage it. Be sure to see your doctor regularly for followup visits.

You also may need certain medications or special procedures. This section explains these treatments and how each can help to protect your heart health.

Medications

Some medications may be used to treat a risk factor for heart disease complications, such as high blood pressure or high blood cholesterol. Others may be prescribed to prevent or relieve the symptoms of heart disease. If you do take medicine, it's important to keep up your heart healthy lifestyle because healthy daily habits will keep your dose of medicine as low as possible. Medications that are commonly prescribed for people with heart disease include:

ACE inhibitors stop the body from producing a chemical that narrows blood vessels. They are used to treat high blood pressure and damaged heart muscle. ACE inhibitors may reduce the risks of a future heart attack and heart failure. They also can prevent kidney damage in some people with diabetes.

Anticoagulants decrease the ability of the blood to clot, and therefore help to prevent clots from forming in your arteries and blocking blood flow. (These medicines are sometimes called blood thinners, though they do not actually thin the blood.) Anticoagulants will not

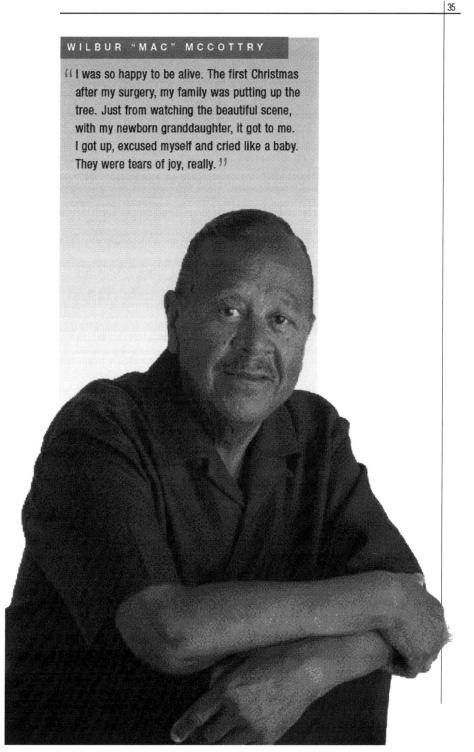

WILBUR "MAC" MCCOTTRY

"I was so happy to be alive. The first Christmas after my surgery, my family was putting up the tree. Just from watching the beautiful scene, with my newborn granddaughter, it got to me. I got up, excused myself and cried like a baby. They were tears of joy, really."

dissolve clots that have already formed, but they may prevent the clots from becoming larger and causing more serious problems.

Antiplatelets are medications that stop blood particles called platelets from clumping together to form harmful clots. These medications may be given to people who have had a heart attack, have angina, or who experience chest pain after an angioplasty procedure. Aspirin is one type of antiplatelet medicine. (See "Aspirin: Take With Caution," on the next page.)

Beta blockers slow the heart rate and allow it to beat with less force. They are used to treat high blood pressure and some arrhythmias (abnormal heart rhythms), and to prevent a repeat heart attack. They can also delay or prevent the development of angina.

Calcium-channel blockers relax blood vessels. They are used to treat high blood pressure, angina, and some arrhythmias.

Cholesterol-lowering drugs are usually used to decrease LDL, or "bad" cholesterol, levels in the blood. Sometimes they are also used to increase HDL, or "good" cholesterol, and to lower triglycerides. Commonly used cholesterol-lowering medications include statins, bile acid sequestrants, niacin, fibrates, and cholesterol-absorption inhibitors.

Digitalis makes the heart contract harder and is used when the heart can't pump strongly enough on its own. It also slows down some fast heart rhythms.

Diuretics (water pills) decrease fluid buildup in the body and are very effective in treating high blood pressure. In addition, new research suggests that diuretics can help to prevent stroke, heart attack, and heart failure. For those who already have heart failure, diuretics can help to reduce fluid buildup in the lungs and swelling in the feet and ankles.

Nitrates relax blood vessels and are used to treat chest pain. Nitrates in different forms can be used to relieve the pain of an angina attack, to prevent an expected episode, or to reduce the number of attacks that occur by using the medicine regularly on a long-term basis. The most commonly used nitrate for angina is nitroglycerin. (See "New Guidelines for Nitroglycerin Use" on page 41.)

Aspirin:
Take With **Caution**

This well-known "wonder drug" is an antiplatelet medicine that can help to lower the risk of a heart attack or stroke for those who have already had one. Aspirin also can help to keep arteries open in those who have had a heart bypass or other artery-opening procedure, such as angioplasty. In addition, aspirin is given to people who arrive at the hospital with a suspected heart attack or stroke.

It's important to know that aspirin has not been approved by the U.S. Food and Drug Administration for the prevention of heart attacks in those who have never had a heart attack or stroke.

However, a recent, large study has found that among healthy women, taking low-dose aspirin every other day may help to prevent a first stroke, and among women over the age of 65, may also help prevent a first heart attack. If you are considering taking aspirin for this purpose, keep in mind that it is a powerful drug with many side effects, and can mix dangerously with other drugs. Take daily aspirin to prevent heart attack only with your doctor's specific advice and guidance. If aspirin is a good choice for you, be sure to take the dose recommended by your doctor.

Antibiotics Aren't the Answer
for Heart Disease Patients

The common bacteria Chlamydia pneumoniae has been found in the arteries of many people with heart disease. In response, some doctors have begun to prescribe antibiotics to their heart patients in the hope that the drug will kill the bug and thereby cut the risk of future heart attacks and other cardiac events.

But new research shows that antibiotics are not effective heart medicines. In two studies involving more than 8,000 people with heart disease, half of the group took an antibiotic regularly for a year or more, while the other group took a placebo, or "sugar pill," that had no biological effect. Nearly 4 years later, the number of heart attacks, strokes, hospitalizations, additional heart procedures, and deaths from heart disease was almost identical between the groups.

The bottom line: Proven treatments, such as lifestyle changes and medications, still offer the best protection against heart attack and other complications of heart disease.

Managing Angina

Angina is chest pain or discomfort caused by a temporary lack of oxygen to the heart muscle. If you have this condition, it's important to manage it well in order to prevent a heart attack and other complications. Here is what you need to know:

Try to avoid triggers. Anything that makes the heart work harder can cause angina pain. Common triggers include certain types of physical activity, emotional stress, cold weather, eating a big meal, high blood pressure, overweight, and cigarette smoking. With the exception of regular, routine physical activity (see "Exercise Safely," page 43), avoid as many of these triggers as you can. Be especially careful to avoid combining triggers, such as going out in cold weather right after eating a heavy meal. You should also avoid heavy lifting and holding your breath when pulling or lifting, since they make your heart work harder.

Don't Forget Your Pills!

"Take your medicine." It sounds simple, but there can be a lot to remember when you take regular medication—especially if you're using more than one. To make the process easier, try these tips:

- Place "sticky notes" in visible places to remind yourself to take your medicines. You might put a note on the fridge, on the bathroom mirror, or on the inside of your front door.
- Use a weekly pill box with separate compartments, available at most drugstores. Keep the box on your kitchen counter or another place where you'll see it frequently throughout the day.
- Use a pill calendar or drug reminder chart. Many doctors' offices make them available to patients on request.
- Wear a wristwatch with an alarm.
- If you use a computer daily, program a startup reminder to take your medicines, or sign up with a free service that will send you a daily reminder e-mail.

Pills

Exercise safely. Certain kinds of exercise can bring on an angina episode. But other, gentler forms of physical activity can actually help to improve your heart health. Getting regular physical activity is a vital part of living well with angina. Talk with your doctor about a safe program of physical activity for you. Participating in a cardiac rehabilitation program is another good way to establish a safe and healthful exercise regimen.

Keep an angina diary. It is important to recognize changes in your angina pattern, including changes in the frequency, length, and severity of episodes. Whenever you notice a change, report it to your doctor right away. To help you keep track of changes, it can help to keep an "angina diary." Using an ordinary notebook, jot down a record of the following:

Prescription for Success:
How To Take Medicines Safely and Effectively

- Before you start any new medicine, give your doctor a list of all of the medications you're already taking, including over-the-counter drugs and supplements. Even better, bring all of your medications to your appointment. This will help your doctor prescribe heart medications that do not mix dangerously with any other medicine you use.
- Take all medicines exactly as your doctor has advised you.
- If you have side effects, tell your doctor right away so that the drugs can be adjusted.
- If you're worried about costs, tell your doctor or pharmacist. There may be a less expensive drug or a generic form that you can use instead.
- Before starting any new over-the-counter medicine or supplement, consult with your doctor or pharmacist to be sure it won't interfere with your prescribed medicine.
- Always get your prescriptions filled on time, so you don't run out. Make a regular note on your calendar to help you remember when to order and pick them up each time.
- Never stop or cut down on any medication without first consulting your doctor.

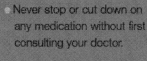

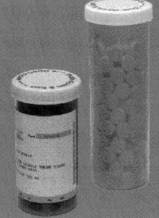

New Guidelines for
Nitroglycerin Use

If you use nitroglycerin to relieve angina symptoms, you probably already know to take a dose promptly whenever you have chest pain or discomfort. Your doctor may have advised you to take up to three doses at 5-minute intervals before calling for emergency help. But new medical guidelines can better protect you from a heart attack. Talk with your doctor about these new recommendations:

- When you experience chest discomfort or pain, place one nitroglycerin tablet under your tongue. (If you use the spray form of the medicine, use one dose of spray.)
- Sit in a comfortable chair or lie down. It is important to rest. If your chest discomfort or pain doesn't improve within 5 minutes, or if it gets worse, call 9–1–1 immediately.
- Even if your chest discomfort goes away within 5 minutes, notify your doctor of the episode.

Nitroglycerin

- The date and time of your discomfort, and how long it lasted
- The trigger or triggers that brought on an episode
- The type and severity of discomfort
- What action you took that relieved your angina

Keep your medicine handy. If you are taking nitroglycerin for angina, it is important to keep it with you at all times. The bottles are very small and can easily be carried in a purse or pocket. Also, be sure to keep the medicine in its original bottle. Get your prescription refilled every 6 months, even if you haven't used up all of the tablets. (Also see above, "New Guidelines for Nitroglycerin Use.")

Procedures

Advanced heart disease may require special procedures to open an artery and improve blood flow. These operations are usually done to ease severe chest pain or clear blood vessel blockages. They include:

Coronary Angioplasty, or "Balloon" Angioplasty
In this procedure, a thin tube called a catheter is threaded through an artery into the narrowed heart vessel. The catheter has a tiny balloon at its tip, which is repeatedly inflated and deflated to open and stretch the artery. Then the balloon is deflated and the catheter removed. This process improves blood flow, reducing chest pain and helping to prevent a heart attack.

Compared with coronary bypass surgery (see page 44), the advantages of angioplasty are that the procedure is less invasive, the patient receives local anesthesia only, and the recovery period is shorter. The disadvantage is that in some cases, the artery closes up again. If this happens, you will need a second angioplasty or bypass surgery.

In most cases, coronary angioplasty is a planned procedure. But it is also used as an emergency treatment during a heart attack to quickly open a blocked coronary artery. The procedure minimizes damage during a heart attack and restores blood flow to the heart muscle.

Plaque Removal
Plaque is the buildup of cholesterol, fat, and other substances in an artery's inner lining. Several procedures have been developed to remove harmful plaque from arteries. In a procedure called an **atherectomy,** a catheter with a rotating shaver on its tip is inserted into an artery to cut away plaque. Another plaque-removal technique is **laser angioplasty,** in which a catheter with a laser at its tip is threaded into an artery where it vaporizes the plaque. Each of these procedures may be used alone or with coronary angioplasty.

Stent Placement
A stent is a tiny wire mesh tube that is used to prop open an artery. A stent is commonly used along with angioplasty and/or plaque removal. In this procedure, a stent is placed over a balloon catheter and then moved into the area of the blockage. When the balloon is inflated, the stent expands and locks into place, holding open the artery. The stent remains in the artery permanently, improving blood flow to the heart muscle and relieving chest pain.

A stent reduces the chances that an artery will narrow again after an angioplasty and/or plaque removal. Newer types of stents are coated with medication that is slowly released and helps to keep the blood vessel from closing up again.

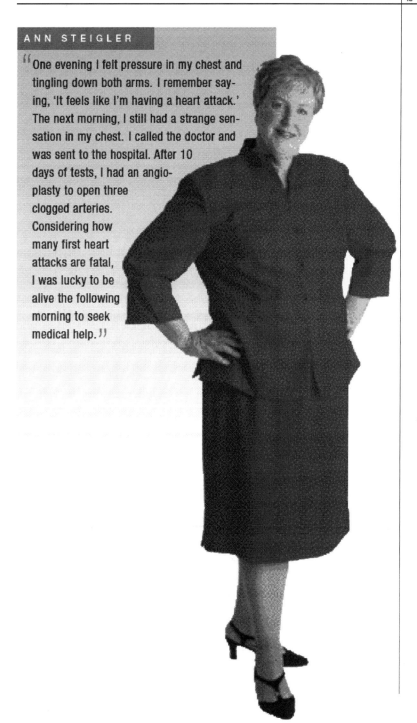

ANN STEIGLER

"One evening I felt pressure in my chest and tingling down both arms. I remember saying, 'It feels like I'm having a heart attack.' The next morning, I still had a strange sensation in my chest. I called the doctor and was sent to the hospital. After 10 days of tests, I had an angioplasty to open three clogged arteries. Considering how many first heart attacks are fatal, I was lucky to be alive the following morning to seek medical help."

Stenting may be particularly beneficial for women. In a large study of heart attack patients, women who received a stent were less likely to suffer a major heart complication during the following year, and also less likely to need a repeat procedure than those who received balloon angioplasty without stenting.

Coronary Bypass Surgery

Bypass surgery is often chosen when artery blockages are hard to reach or are too extensive for angioplasty. In this procedure, the surgeon takes a piece of blood vessel from the leg or chest and then attaches it to the heart artery both above and below the narrowed area. This procedure creates a new route, or "bypass," around the blockage. Afterward, the blood can use this new pathway to flow freely to the heart muscle, thereby reducing the risk of a heart attack. In some cases, more than one bypass is necessary.

For most operations, the patient is connected to a heart-lung machine that delivers oxygen to the blood and circulates blood throughout the body so that the heart can be temporarily stopped while the bypass is made. When the surgery is finished, the heart is restarted. A person who undergoes bypass surgery usually stays in the hospital for about a week, and then continues to recuperate for several weeks at home.

Two recently developed types of bypass surgery do not require use of the heart-lung machine. They are:

Off-pump coronary bypass. In this procedure, the heart is kept beating and just the portion of the heart with the affected artery is held still while the bypass graft is sewn into place. While more study is needed on this approach, recent research suggests that this type of bypass surgery may have fewer complications than conventional bypass surgery, particularly for overweight and elderly patients.

Minimally invasive coronary artery bypass. This procedure is intended for use only when one or two arteries will be bypassed. Also performed while the heart is still beating, the surgery uses a combination of small holes in the chest and a small incision made directly over the artery to be bypassed. The surgeon usually detaches an artery from inside the chest wall and reattaches it to the clogged artery furthest away from the blockage. This operation usually has a shorter recovery time than conventional bypass surgery.

Implantable Defibrillators:
New Hope for
Heart Failure Patients

An implantable cardiac defibrillator (ICD) is a small, battery-powered device that uses an electric signal to automatically correct an abnormal heartbeat. Implanted beneath the skin of the chest, ICDs have been used during the past decade to treat life-threatening arrhythmias. Now, new research suggests that an implantable defibrillator can help to extend the lives of people with heart failure.

About 50 percent of deaths in heart failure are sudden deaths that are probably due to an abnormally fast heartbeat in one of the heart's lower chambers. In a large study of patients with moderate to severe heart failure, one-third of participants were treated with an implantable defibrillator, while one-third took the anti-arrhythmia drug amiodarone (sold as Cordarone or Pacerone), and another one-third received neither treatment. The results: ICD treatment significantly reduced deaths over the next 4 years, while the medication did not. The benefit from ICD therapy appeared to be strongest among those with moderate heart failure.

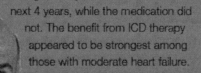

Defibrillators

Getting Help for a Heart Attack

For many people, the first symptom of heart disease is a heart attack. That means everyone should know how to identify the symptoms of a heart attack and how to get immediate medical help. Ideally, treatment should start within 1 hour of the first symptoms. Recognizing the warning signs and getting help quickly can save your life.

Know the Warning Signs

Not all heart attacks begin with sudden, crushing pain, as is often shown on TV or in the movies. Many heart attacks start slowly with mild pain or discomfort. The most common warning signs are:

- **Chest discomfort.** Most heart attacks involve discomfort in the center of the chest that lasts for more than a few minutes. It may feel like uncomfortable pressure, squeezing, fullness, or pain. The discomfort can be mild or severe, and it may come and go.
- **Discomfort in other areas of the upper body,** including one or both arms, the back, neck, jaw, or stomach.
- **Shortness of breath.** This symptom may occur with or without chest discomfort.
- **Other signs include nausea,** light-headedness, or breaking out in a cold sweat.

Get Help Quickly

If you think that you or someone else may be having a heart attack, you must act quickly to prevent disability or death, and to get the most benefit from current treatments. Wait no more than a few minutes—5 at most—before calling 9–1–1.

It is important to call 9–1–1 because emergency medical personnel can begin treatment even before you get to the hospital. They also have the equipment and training to start your heart beating again if it stops. Calling 9–1–1 quickly can save your life.

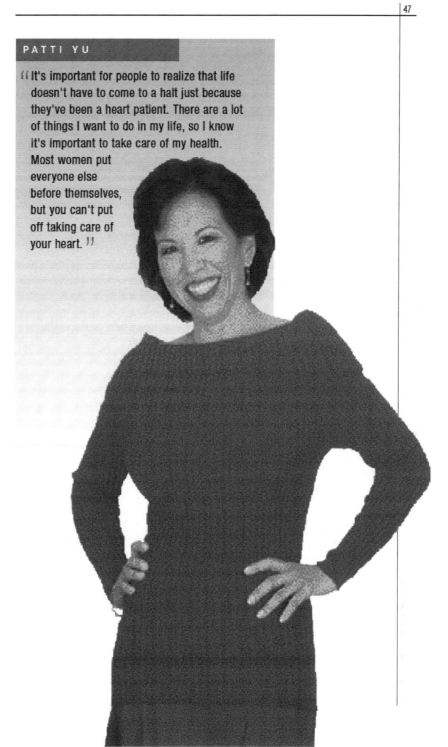

PATTI YU

"It's important for people to realize that life doesn't have to come to a halt just because they've been a heart patient. There are a lot of things I want to do in my life, so I know it's important to take care of my health. Most women put everyone else before themselves, but you can't put off taking care of your heart."

Even if you're not sure you're having a heart attack, call 9–1–1 if your symptoms last up to 5 minutes. If your symptoms stop completely in less than 5 minutes, you should still call your doctor right away.

You must also act at once because hospitals have clot-dissolving medicines and other artery-opening treatments that can stop a heart attack if given quickly. These treatments work best when given within the first hour after a heart attack starts.

When you get to the hospital, don't be afraid to speak up for what you need—or bring someone who can speak up for you. Ask for tests that can determine if you are having a heart attack. Commonly given initial tests include an electrocardiogram (EKG or ECG) and a cardiac blood test (to check for heart damage). You have the right to be thoroughly examined for a possible heart attack. If you are having a heart attack, you have the right to immediate treatment to help stop the attack.

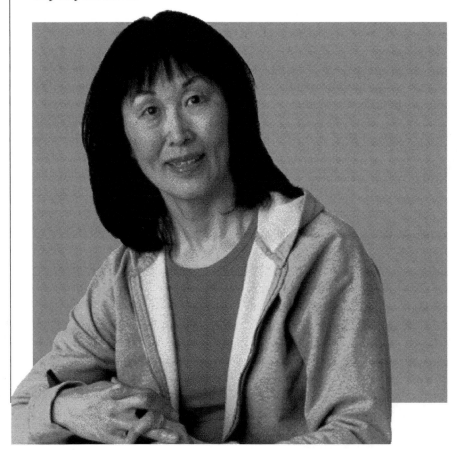

Plan Ahead

Nobody plans on having a heart attack. But just as many people have a plan in case of fire, it is important to make a plan to deal with a possible heart attack. Taking the following steps can preserve your health—and your life.

- Learn the heart attack warning signs "by heart."
- Talk with family and friends about the warning signs and the need to call 9–1–1 quickly.
- Talk with your doctor about your risk factors for heart attack and how to reduce them.
- Write out a "heart attack survival plan" that includes important medical information and keep it handy. (Use the accompanying box on page 50 as a guide.)
- Arrange in advance to have someone else care for your children or other dependents in an emergency.

Delay Can Be Deadly

Most people who have a heart attack wait too long to seek medical help—and that can be a fatal mistake. Some delay because they don't understand the symptoms of a heart attack and think that what they're feeling is due to something else. Others put off getting help because they don't want to worry others or "cause a scene," especially if their symptoms turn out to be a false alarm. Women are especially likely to delay. A large study of heart attack patients found that, on average, women waited 22 minutes longer than men did before going to the hospital.

Don't wait. When you're facing something as serious as a possible heart attack, it's much better to be safe than sorry. Waiting too long can cause permanent disability or death. If you have any symptoms of a possible heart attack that last up to 5 minutes, call 9–1–1 right away.

Don't Delay

Heart Attack Survival Plan

Fill out the form below and make several copies. Keep one copy near your home phone, where you can easily see it. Keep another copy at work, and a third copy in your wallet or purse.

Information To Share With Emergency Medical Personnel and Hospital Staff

Medicines you are taking:

_____
_____
_____
_____
_____

Medicines you are allergic to:

_____
_____
_____
_____
_____

How To Contact Your Doctor
If symptoms stop completely in less than 5 minutes, you should still call your doctor right away.

Phone number during office hours:_____
Phone number after office hours:_____

Person To Contact If You Go to the Hospital

Name:_____
Home phone number:_____
Work phone number:_____

Survival Plan

Recovering Well: Life After a Heart Attack or Heart Procedure

Having a heart attack or a heart procedure can be a frightening and upsetting experience. It is difficult to discover—often suddenly—that your body isn't working the way it should, and to be plunged into an unfamiliar world of hospitals and high-tech procedures. But it's important to know that millions of people have survived a heart attack, recovered fully, and gone on to resume active, normal lives. Likewise, most people who undergo heart surgery recover well and return to their usual activities. Many surgery patients eventually feel healthier than they did before their procedure.

The time it takes to get back to normal will depend on many factors, including your age and general health. If you have had a heart attack, the pace of recovery will also depend on the severity of the attack. If you have undergone surgery, recovery time will depend partly on the type of procedure you had. But whatever your situation, there is much you can do to

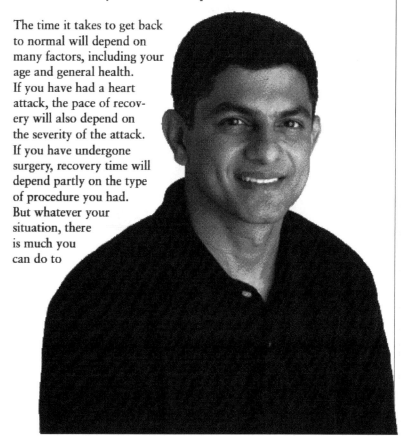

improve your health and prevent complications following a heart attack or major heart procedure.

The first step: Give yourself permission to recover. You and your body have been through a lot, and it will take some time to feel like yourself again. Expect to feel quite tired at first, and to gradually regain your strength and energy. While individual needs vary, following are some overall tips for recovering well from a heart attack or heart surgery.

Your First Weeks at Home

When you first arrive home from the hospital, you'll need to get a lot of rest so that your heart can begin to heal. It is very important to eat healthfully and to get enough sleep. Take the medications your doctor has prescribed for you. (See "Heart-Healing Medicines" on the next page.) Avoid heavy yard work, house cleaning, or other projects that require a lot of energy. Also refrain from physical activity in very hot or cold weather. Ask family and friends to help out with chores, childcare, and other activities that may be difficult to take care of during your first weeks at home.

At the same time, it is important to get up and move around as you begin to recover. Your heart is a muscle that needs be exercised— though very gently at first. Pace yourself. Allow plenty of time for each thing you do during the day, from getting out of bed to taking a shower to preparing a simple breakfast. Rest between activities, and whenever you feel tired. Ask your doctor for a list of guidelines for activity during your first few weeks at home.

Your doctor will want to check your progress 1 to 4 weeks after you leave the hospital. During your first followup visit, your doctor will check your weight and blood pressure, make any needed changes in your medicines, perform necessary tests, and check how your recovery is progressing overall. Use this opportunity to ask any questions you may have about safe or unsafe activities, medicines, lifestyle changes, or any other issues that concern you. You may want to write down your questions beforehand.

For some situations and questions, it is best to call your doctor right away rather than wait for your next appointment. Call promptly if:

Heart-Healing Medicines

Following a heart attack, your doctor will probably prescribe one or more drugs to improve your heart functioning and help prevent another heart attack. If your doctor doesn't mention medicine, ask whether you should take one of the following medications. (For more information on the purpose and impact of each drug, see the more detailed "Medications" section on pages 38–40.)

- ACE inhibitors
- Aspirin
- Beta blockers
- LDL cholesterol-lowering and triglyceride-lowering drugs

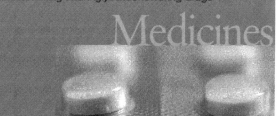

- You have symptoms related to your original heart disease, such as trouble breathing, chest pain, weakness, or an irregular heartbeat.
- You notice side effects after starting a new heart medicine.
- You've been given a prescription for a condition other than heart disease. It is important to find out whether it's safe to take other medicines along with your heart drugs.
- You've recently had heart surgery or another kind of medical treatment and you notice symptoms that your doctor has warned you about.
- You feel down or "have the blues" for more than a few days.

If you have symptoms of a possible heart attack, call 9–1–1 right away. See pages 46–50 for the warning signs of a heart attack and how to act fast to get help.

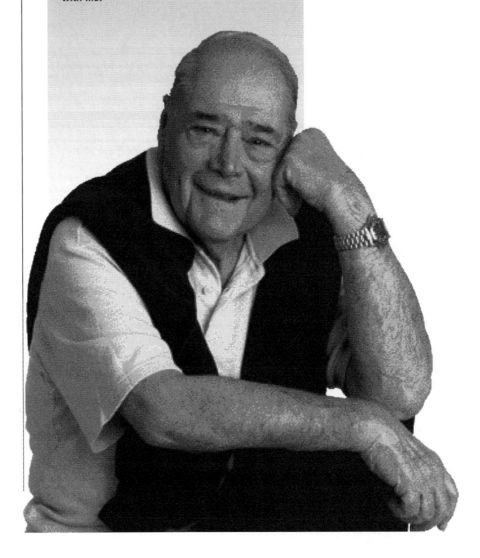

BOB GELENTER

"I was diagnosed with an enlarged heart, had heart surgery and now have a pacemaker. I have learned that if you have a chronic disease, it does not mean you have a terminal disease. You can live with heart disease. Since my surgery, I've been working on losing weight. My wife helps me by getting workout tapes from the library and doing the exercises with me."

Cardiac Rehabilitation

Your doctor may recommend cardiac rehabilitation (rehab) to help you recover from a heart attack or heart surgery. This is a total program for heart health that includes exercise training, education on heart healthy living, and counseling to reduce stress and help you return to an active life.

Getting involved in a cardiac rehab program is an excellent idea. A recent study showed that people who participated in cardiac rehab were 50 percent more likely to survive 3 years after a heart attack than those who didn't participate. Cardiac rehab can help to strengthen your heart, reduce the risks of a future heart attack, and return you as quickly as possible to your normal daily activities. Almost everyone with heart disease can benefit from some kind of cardiac rehabilitation. No one is too old or too young to benefit. Women are helped by cardiac rehab as much as men are.

Getting Started

Cardiac rehab often begins in the hospital after a heart attack or heart surgery, with very gentle physical activity and counseling on adjusting to life at home. Once you leave the hospital, you can continue to participate in cardiac rehab on an outpatient basis. Outpatient programs may be located at your hospital, in a medical center, or in a community facility such as a YMCA. Some people continue cardiac rehabilitation at home. Regardless of the location, your cardiac rehab team—which may include doctors, nurses, exercise specialists, dietitians and counselors—will help you to create a safe exercise plan, as well as provide information and encouragement to control your risk factors.

You will need your doctor's approval to get started in cardiac rehab. But not all doctors bring up the topic with their heart patients, especially women. Research indicates that women are only about half as likely as men to participate in cardiac rehab programs. This is worrisome, because nonparticipation increases the risk of having second and often fatal heart attacks. So be sure to tell your doctor or nurse that you're interested in cardiac rehabilitation. Talk with them about your specific needs and preferences, and ask for a referral that is a good fit for you.

How To Choose a Cardiac Rehab Program

Cardiac rehab programs vary in the types of services they offer and emphasize. Choose one that makes exercise training a priority. Studies show that people who participate in an exercise-based program are less likely to have a future heart attack or major heart surgery, and are less apt to die of any heart-related cause than those who don't join a program that emphasizes exercise. When choosing a cardiac rehab program, also look for one that:

- Offers a wide range of services, including education and counseling.
- Offers services at a time and place that are convenient for you.
- Offers services that meet your specific needs and preferences. For example, if you're overweight, look for a plan that provides help for weight loss.
- Is supervised by a team of health care professionals.
- Is affordable. Your insurance may cover the cost of some cardiac rehab services, but not others. Find out what will be covered and for how long, so you'll know from the start what your out-of-pocket costs will be.

What You'll Do in a Cardiac Rehab Program

Get moving. Exercise training will help you learn to safely participate in physical activity, strengthen your muscles, and improve your stamina. If you've recently gotten out of the hospital, you may be worried that exercise will bring on another heart attack or other heart crisis. In fact, physical activity can help prevent future heart problems. Your rehab team will help you develop a program that is safe and effective for you.

Some programs make use of equipment such as a treadmill for walking, stationary bikes, and light weights, and you'll be shown how to use this equipment to get the most benefit. Other programs offer low-impact aerobics classes and other group exercise activities. In most programs, your heart rate and blood pressure will be monitored while you move. As your heart and body become stronger, you will gradually increase your physical activity. Eventually, after you become familiar with the program, you can continue it at a fitness center or at home.

Learn new heart healthy habits. In your cardiac rehab program, you'll also learn about controlling your personal risk factors for heart attack and other heart complications, and how to create new, healthier habits. Controlling risk factors is a very important part of your recovery process. Depending on your personal needs, you may learn to:

- Quit smoking if you're a smoker.
- Manage related health conditions such as diabetes and high blood pressure.
- Eat a healthy, low-saturated fat, low-cholesterol diet.
- Control your weight.
- Manage stress.

For more information on controlling risk factors, see the sections of this guidebook on "Major Risk Factors" and "What Else Affects Heart Disease?" on pages 13 and 31 respectively.

Get counseling and support. A good cardiac rehab program will help you learn to cope with the challenges of adjusting to a new lifestyle, as well as address any concerns you may have about the future. You'll also be offered help in dealing with the emotional ups and downs that many people experience following a heart attack or heart surgery. Many programs offer classes in stress management, as well individual counseling, group support, or both.

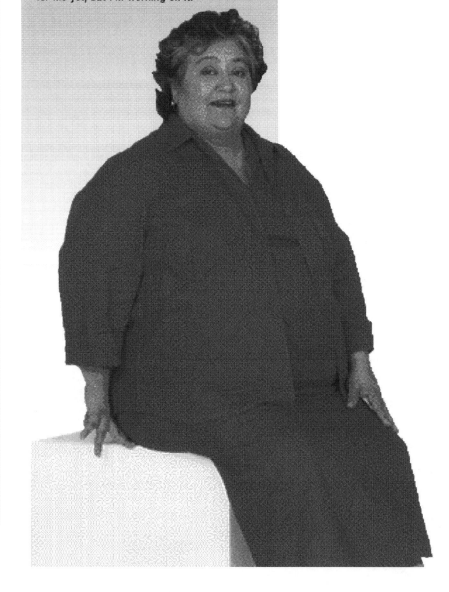

BALERMA BURGESS

" I know that if I don't change things in my life, I might not live to see my grandchildren. Every day, I talk myself into doing things for my health, like taking the stairs instead of the elevator and eating more fruits and vegetables. These things haven't become habits for me yet, but I'm working on it. "

Getting the Most Out of Cardiac Rehab
You'll benefit most from your cardiac rehab program by becoming as actively involved in it as possible. Think of yourself as the most important member of your recovery team—because you are. Join with health care professionals in designing or adjusting services to best meet your needs. Show up for exercise, education, and support sessions. Ask questions. Report any changes in your feelings or symptoms.

Finally, be sure to complete the program. Even if you feel that you already "have a handle" on how to recover, keep in mind that your needs will continue to change throughout the recovery process. Your cardiac rehab team can help you respond to those changing needs, and thereby continue to help you improve your heart health. So stick with the program!

Getting Your Life Back

As you begin to recover from a heart attack or heart procedure, you may naturally wonder when you can return to your usual activities, including work, sexual activity, driving, and travel. Most people can safely return to most of their normal activities within a few weeks, as long as they do not have chest pain or other complications. While you should ask your doctor when you can return to each of your usual activities, here are some general guidelines:

Work. Most people are able to return to their usual work within several weeks. Your doctor may ask you to take tests to find out if you can do the kind of job you did before. While most individuals can continue their customary work with no problems, some people choose to change jobs or reduce their hours to lighten the load on their heart. Counselors at cardiac rehab programs may be able to provide support and resources for those considering a job change.

Sexual activity. Most people can have sexual relations again about 3–6 weeks after a heart attack or heart procedure, as long they have no chest pain or other complications. But since everyone recovers at his or her own pace, your doctor may give you a stress test to determine when you can safely resume sexual activity. When you're ready for sex again, choose a time when you feel relaxed and rested. Wait at least an hour after eating a full meal to allow time for digestion. Take your time. If you have chest pain or other heart symptoms during sexual activity, have lost interest, or are worried about having sex, talk with your doctor.

A special note: Couples who use medication to enhance sex should know that these drugs can cause irregular heartbeats. If you've been using one of these medicines or are considering taking one, ask your doctor whether it is safe to do so.

Driving can usually begin within a week for most patients, if allowed by State law. Each State has its own regulations for driving a motor vehicle following a serious illness, so contact your State's Department of Motor Vehicles for guidelines. People with complications or chest pain should not drive until their symptoms have been stable for a few weeks.

Travel. Once your doctor tells you it's safe for you to travel, keep these tips in mind:

- Keep your medications in your purse or carry-on luggage so they will be easily available when you need them.
- Pack light so that you can lift your luggage without strain. At the airport, train, or bus station, use a pull-cart to cut down on lifting. If possible, get help from a porter.
- Allow more time than usual to catch your flight, train, or bus. Who needs the extra stress?
- Walk around at least every 2 hours during trips. While sitting, flex your feet frequently and do other simple exercises to increase blood flow in your legs and prevent blood clots.
- Check with your doctor before traveling to locations at high altitudes (greater than 6,000 feet) or places where the temperature will be either very hot or very cold. When you first arrive, give yourself a chance to rest.

Remember, each person's recovery process is different. Don't try to guess when you can return to normal activities. Always ask your doctor first.

Coping With Your Feelings

Anyone who has had a heart attack or has undergone heart surgery knows that it can be an upsetting experience. You've just come through a major health crisis, and your usual life has been disrupted. Afterward, it's normal to experience a wide range of feelings. You

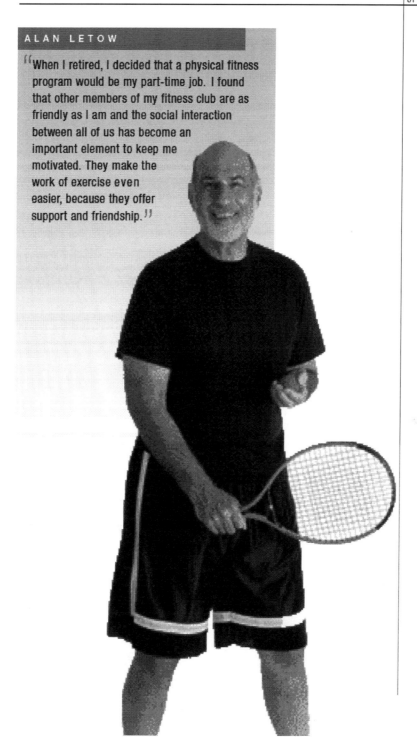

ALAN LETOW

"When I retired, I decided that a physical fitness program would be my part-time job. I found that other members of my fitness club are as friendly as I am and the social interaction between all of us has become an important element to keep me motivated. They make the work of exercise even easier, because they offer support and friendship."

may feel some relief. But you may also feel worried, angry, or depressed. It may be reassuring to know that these reactions are very common, and that most difficult feelings pass within a few weeks. Here are some things to remember:

Take 1 day at a time. Try not to think too much about next week or next month. Do what you can do today. Enjoy small pleasures: a walk in your neighborhood, a conversation with a loved one, a snuggle with a pet, or a good meal.

Share your concerns. Talk with family members and friends about your feelings and concerns, and ask for support. Be sure to ask for the kind of support you need. (For example, if you want a sympathetic ear rather than advice, gently let your loved ones know.) Be sure to give family members time to say what they feel and need, too. Supportive relationships may actually help to lengthen life after a heart attack.

Get support from "veterans." Whether you've had a heart attack or gone through heart surgery, consider joining a support group for people who have shared your experience. Groups for heart patients can provide emotional support as well as help you develop new ways of handling everyday challenges. For a list of support groups in your local area, contact The Mended Hearts at www.mended.hearts.org or at 1–888–432–7899. Your local American Heart Association chapter may also offer support groups.

Keep moving. Regular physical activity not only helps to reduce the risk of future heart problems, but also helps to relieve anxiety, depression, and other difficult feelings. Any regular physical activity—even gentle walking—can help to lift your mood.

Seek help for depression. Up to 20 percent of heart disease patients battle serious depression, and many more suffer milder cases of the "blues." If you find yourself feeling very sad or discouraged for more than a week or so, be sure to let your doctor know. Counseling and/or medication can often be very helpful. Seeking help is very important, not only because you deserve to enjoy life as fully as possible, but also because heart patients who are successfully treated for depression are less likely to have future serious heart problems.

Caring for Your Heart

There's no getting around it: Heart disease changes your life. For many people, living with a heart condition requires changes both big and small, from undergoing major surgery to adding more fruits and vegetables to their diets. Change can be difficult, and sometimes even scary. But with support, resources, and a good supply of determination, most people are able to meet these new challenges well.

So pick up this book whenever you need it for information and encouragement. Ask for support from family and friends. Keep in touch with your doctor. Make new, heart healthy lifestyle choices, one healthful habit at a time.

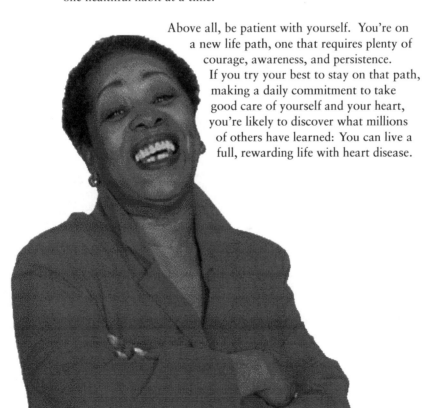

Above all, be patient with yourself. You're on a new life path, one that requires plenty of courage, awareness, and persistence. If you try your best to stay on that path, making a daily commitment to take good care of yourself and your heart, you're likely to discover what millions of others have learned: You can live a full, rewarding life with heart disease.

To Learn More

The National Heart, Lung, and Blood Institute provides information on the prevention and treatment of heart disease and offers publications on heart health and heart disease.

NHLBI Health Information Center
P.O. Box 30105
Bethesda, MD 20824-0105
Phone: 301–592–8573
TTY: 240–629–3255
Fax: 301–592–8563

NHLBI Heart Health Information Line
1–800–575–WELL
Provides toll-free recorded messages.

Also, check out these heart health Web sites and Web pages:

NHLBI Web site: www.nhlbi.nih.gov

Diseases and Conditions A–Z Index:
http://www.nhlbi.nih.gov/health/dci/index.html

The Heart Truth: A National Awareness Campaign for Women About Heart Disease: www.hearttruth.gov

Your Guide to Lowering High Blood Pressure:
www.nhlbi.nih.gov/hbp/index.html

Live Healthier, Live Longer (on lowering elevated blood cholesterol):
www.nhlbi.nih.gov/chd

High Blood Cholesterol: What You Need To Know:
www.nhlbi.nih.gov/health/public/heart/chol/hbc_what.htm

Aim for a Healthy Weight:
www.nhlbi.nih.gov/health/public/heart/obesity/lose_wt/index.htm

Act in Time to Heart Attack Signs:
www.nhlbi.nih.gov/actintime/index.htm

Heart Healthy Recipes:
www.nhlbi.nih.gov/health/public/heart/other/syah/index.htm
http://www.nhlbi.nih.gov/health/public/heart/other/ktb_recipebk/

Smoking Cessation: For information from the National Cancer Institute on quitting smoking, call 1–800–QUITNOW
(1–800–784–8669) or go to http://www.smokefree.gov/

For still more information on heart health, see Medline Plus:
http://medlineplus.gov/

Made in the USA
Las Vegas, NV
01 March 2022

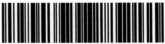

44828078R00039